PAGE *
MERGEFO
RMAT

96

STROKE RECOVERY

A complete guide on Stroke, Types, Risk factors, Medical prescriptions and possible cure: Also a guide for care givers, patients, & health professionals.

Dr. Kate D. Martins (Ph.D)

PREFACE

If you enjoy this book, please leave a review.

Also send me your thoughts about this book including the errors or what needs to be added via this mail: will394560@gmail.com in return you will get a FREE copy of my next book.

TABLE OF CONTENT

INTRODUCTION

THE HISTORY OF STROKE

Episodes of stroke and familial stroke was reported consistently from the second thousand years (millennium) BC ahead in Ancient Persia and Mesotopia. Hippocrates (460 to 370 BC) was first to portray the peculiarity and phenomenon of sudden paralysis that is frequently connected with ischemia.

The word Apoplexy, which was gotten from the Greek word signifying "struck down with violence", first showed in Hippocratic writings to depict this phenomenon. The word stroke was used more as a synonym for motionless and apoplectic seizure in the year 1599, and is the literal interpretation of the Greek term or expression. The term apoplectic stroke is an old, vague term, for a cerebrovascular accident accompanied by haemorrhagic stroke. Martin Luther was depicted and described to have an apoplectic stroke that denied him of his speech shortly before his demise in 1546.

In 1658, in his Apoplexia, Johann Jacob Wepfer (1620-1695) identified the reason for hemorrhagic stroke when he proposed that individuals who had passed on from apoplexy had series of bleeds in their brains. Wepfer likewise identified the principal arteries providing the brain, the vertebral and carotid veins, and found out the cause and reason for a kind of ischemic stroke known as a cerebral infarction when he recommended that apoplexy may be caused by a blockage to those vessels. Rudolf Virchow originally described the component of thromboembolism as a significant and major factor.

AN OVERVIEW OF STROKE

Cerebrovascular as a term, was presented in the year 1927, mirroring a "developing awareness and acknowledgment of vascular hypotheses and a recognition of the outcomes of an unexpected disruption in the vascular stockpile (supply) of the brain". Its use is currently deterred by various nervous system science material (like text books), thinking that the meaning and connotation fortuitousness conveyed by the word accident deficiently features the modifiability of the hidden risk factors.

Brain attack, as a term, was introduced for use with highlight the acute nature of stroke as indicated by the American Stroke Association, which has used the term since the year 1990, and is used conversationally to mean both ischemic as well as hemorrhagic stroke.

Stroke (otherwise called a brain attack or cerebrovascular accident (CVA)) is a condition, (a medical one) where blood stream to the brain causes cell death. There are two principal types of stroke: ischemic, because of insufficient blood flow, and hemorrhagic, Because of bleeding. Both cause portion of the cerebrum (brain) to stop working and functioning properly.

CHAPTER ONE
CLASSIFICATION/ SYMPTOMS

*Stroke can be classified into two significant classes: **Ischemic** and **Hemorrhagic**.*

Ischemic stroke is brought about by interference of the blood supply to the cerebrum, while hemorrhagic stroke results from the rupture of a vein or a strange vascular structure. Around 87% of stroke is ischemic, with the rest being hemorrhagic. It's possible for bleeding to develop inside areas of ischemia, a condition better known as "hemorrhagic change." It is still unknown number of cases of hemorrhagic stroke that really start as ischemic stroke.

DEFINITION

In the year 1970, the WHO (World Health Organization) defined stroke as a "neurological deficiency of cerebrovascular cause that perseveres past 24 hours or is intruded on by death inside 24 hours albeit stroke is extremely old. This definition should mirror the reversibility of tissue harm or damage and was conceived for the reason, with the time span of 24 hours being picked randomly. The 24-hour limit divides stroke from transient ischemic attack, which is a connected condition of stroke symptoms that settle totally inside 24 hours. With the availability of medicines that can diminish stroke severity when given on time, many presently prefer alternative, for example, acute ischemic, brain attack, cerebrovascular disorder (demonstrated after respiratory failure and intense coronary condition), to mirror the urgency of stroke symptoms and the need to act swiftly.

ISCHEMIC

With Ischemic stroke, blood supply to a region of the brain is diminished, prompting to a malfunction of the cerebrum tissue around the region.

There are 4 main reasons as to why this could occur:

- *Apoplexy (hindrance of a vein by a blood coagulation or clot locally)*
- *Embolism (obstruction because of an embolus from somewhere else in the body)*
- *Hypo-perfusion of the system (a gradual and general decrease in blood supply, e.g., in shock)*
- *Cerebral venous sinus thrombosis.*

Stroke without an obvious or regular explanation is named cryptogenic stroke (idiopathic); this comprises 30-40% of ischemic stroke.

There are different and many other classification system for Acute ischemic stroke. The Oxford Community Stroke Project (OCSP), otherwise called the Bamford or Oxford characterization) depends essentially on the initial signs and symptoms; in view of the degree of the symptoms, the stroke episode is classified as total anterior infarct (TACI), posterior circulation infarct (POCI), lacunar infarct (LACI), or partial anterior circulation infarct (PACI).

These four elements determines the degree of the stroke, the region of the brain that is affected, the hidden reason, and the prognosis. The TOAST (Trial of Organization 10172 in acute Stroke Treatment) classification depends on signs and symptoms as well as consequences of additional examinations and investigations; on this premise, stroke is classified as being because of:

(1) A total and complete blockage of a small blood vessel,

(2) Apoplexy or embolism because of atherosclerosis of a very large artery,

(3) An embolism originating in the heart

(4) Various determined causes,

(5) Users of items that stimulate, for example, cocaine and methamphetamine are at great risk for Ischemic stroke.

HEMORRHAGIC

Intracerebral hemorrhage, which is bleeding inside the cerebrum itself (when an artery in the brain explodes, flooding the encompassing tissue with blood), due to intraparenchymal hemorrhage (bleeding inside the cerebrum tissue) or intraventricular hemorrhage (bleeding inside the brains ventricular framework).

Subarachnoid hemorrhage, which is bleeding that happens outside the brain tissue yet inside the skull, and definitively between the arachnoid mater and pia mater (the fragile deepest layer of the three layers of the meninges that encompass the cerebrum).

The 2 main types of hemorrhagic stroke mentioned above likewise two unique forms of intracranial hemorrhage, which is the collection of blood anywhere inside the cranial vault; however different forms of intracranial hemorrhage, like epidural hematoma (bleeding between the dura mater and the skull, which is the thick peripheral layer of the meninges that encompass the brain) and subdural hematoma (bleeding in the subdural space), are not seen as "hemorrhagic stroke".

Hemorrhagic stroke might occur on the foundation of adjustments to the veins in the cerebrum, for example, cerebral amyloid angiopathy, cerebral arteriovenous distortion and an intracranial aneurysm, which can lead to intraparenchymal or subarachnoid hemorrhage.

Notwithstanding neurological impairment, hemorrhagic stroke normally causes certain symptoms (for example, subarachnoid discharge or hemorrhage traditionally causes a serious migraine known as a thunderbolt headache) or uncover proof of a past head injury.

SIGNS AND SIDE EFFECTS

Stroke signs and symptoms normally start abruptly, over seconds then minutes, and as in most cases don't advance further. The signs and symptoms normally rely upon the region of the brain affected. The greater and broader the region of the brain is affected, the more casual and day-to-day capabilities that are probably going to be lost. A few types of stroke can cause extra side effects. For instance, in intracranial hemorrhage, the affected region might compress other systems and structures. Most types of stroke are not related with a migraine (headache), aside from subarachnoid hemorrhage and cerebral venous apoplexy and sometimes intracerebral hemorrhage.

EARLY ACKNOWLEDGMENT

Different systems have been proposed to increase acknowledgment of stroke. Various discoveries can anticipate or predict the presence or absence of stroke to various degrees.

- ☐ *Unexpected beginning face weakness,*
- ☐ *Arm drift (i.e., if an individual, when being asked to raise the two arms,*

automatically allows one arm to fall downwards) and

☐ *Unusual or abnormal speech. These are the discoveries probably going to lead to the right identification of stroke, improving the probability by 5.5 when one of these symptoms is available. Essentially, when every one of the three of these are missing, the probability of stroke is lowered (-probability proportion of 0.39). While these discoveries are not perfect for diagnosing stroke, the way that they can be assessed and evaluated generally quickly and effectively make them truly important in the acute setting.*

For individuals referred to the emergency room, early acknowledgment of stroke is considered significant as this can facilitate symptomatic or diagnostic tests and treatments. A scoring system, ROSIER (acknowledgment of stroke in the emergency room) is suggested for this reason; it depends on features from the physical examination and medical history.

SUBTYPES

Assuming that the region of the brain affected includes one of the three most important central nervous system pathways — the corticospinal tract, spinothalamic tract, and the dorsal column lemniscus pathway, signs and symptoms might include:

- *Numbness*
- *Hemiplegia and muscle weakness of the face*
- *Decrease in vibratory or sensory sensation*
- *Initial flaccidity (lowered muscle tone), supplanted by spasticity (increased muscle tone), extreme reflexes, and compulsory synergies.*

Generally speaking, the symptoms usually affects just a unilateral (one side of the body). Contingent on the part of the brain affected, the problem and defect in the cerebrum (brain) is always usually on the opposite side of the body. Nonetheless, since these pathways likewise travel in the spinal cord and any sore there can likewise develop and produce these very symptoms, but the presence of any of these symptoms doesn't really identifies stroke. Now adding to the central nervous system pathways, the brainstem provides rise to 12 major cranial nerves.

- ☐ *Altered taste, hearing, smell, or vision (partial or total)*
- ☐ *Weakness of ocular muscles and Drooping of eyelid*
- ☐ *Decreased reflexes: gag, pupil reactivity to light, swallow*

- ☐ *Decreased sensation and muscle weakness of the face*
- ☐ *Altered heart and breathing rate*
- ☐ *Problems with balance and nystagmus*
- ☐ *Weakness in sternocleidomastoid muscle also with the in ability to turn head to another side*
- ☐ *Failure and weakness in tongue (inability to stick out the tongue or move it from one side to another)*

In the event that the cerebral cortex is involved, the central nervous system pathways can again be affected, however can likewise deliver the following signs and symptoms:

1. *Aphasia (trouble with verbal articulation or expression, reading and writing, auditory comprehension: Broca's or Wernicke's region usually involved*
2. *Visual field defect*
3. *Dysarthria (motor speech disorder brought about because of neurological injury)*
4. *Hemineglect (involvement of parietal lobe)*
5. *Apraxia (Altered voluntary movements)*
6. *Memory shortfalls (involvement of parietal lobe)*
7. *Disordered or disorganized thinking, hypersexual*

motions, confusion (with association of cerebrum)

8. *Absence of knowledge of his or her, normally stroke-related, disability*

Assuming that the cerebellum is involved, ataxia may be present and this incorporates:

- *Altered movement coordination*
- *Dizziness or potentially disequilibrium*
- *Altered walking gait*

Other Related symptoms include:

Headache, loss of consciousness, and vomiting for the most part happen more frequently in hemorrhagic stroke than in apoplexy in light of the increased intracranial pressure from the liking blood compacting or compressing the brain.

In the event that symptoms are maximal at beginning, the reason is bound to be a subarachnoid hemorrhage or an embolic stroke.

CHAPTER TWO
CAUSES

THROMBOTIC STROKE

In thrombotic stroke, a thrombus (blood cluster or clot) for the most part normally form around atherosclerotic plaques. Since blockage of the artery is usually gradual, the start of thrombotic stroke is slower than that of hemorrhagic stroke. A thrombus itself (regardless of whether it totally block the vein) can prompt an embolic stroke (you will see below) if by any chance the thrombus breaks off and goes in the circulation system (bloodstream), which at some point is called an embolus. 2 types of thrombotic can cause stroke:

Large vessel sickness involves the normal and inside carotid arteries, the vertebral arteries, and the Circle of Willis: *Illnesses that might form thrombi in the large vessels are (in a descending order): atherosclerosis, carotid or vertebral artery dissection, vasoconstriction (tightening of the artery), aortic, inflammatory illnesses of the blood* vessel (Takamasa arteritis, giant cell arteritis), Moyamoya infection, fibromuscular dysplasia, and no inflammatory vasculopthy. Strokes brought about by artery dissection are in the strictest sense not generally brought about by a 'defined disease state', such occasions can happen in young individuals and can be brought about by physical injury, for example, hyperextension of the neck region or by different types of trauma.

Small vessel sickness involves the smaller veins inside the cerebrum: parts of the circle of Willis, middle cerebral artery, stem, and arteries arising from the distal vertebral and basilar artery. Illnesses that might develop thrombi in the small vessels include (in descending other): lipohyalinosis (development of fatty hyaline matter in the vein because of hypertension, pressure and aging) and fibrinoid degeneration (stroke *including these vessels is known as a lacunar stroke) and micro-atheroma (small atherosclerotic plaques).*

Iron deficiency (Anemia) causes increment blood flow in the blood circulatory system. This makes the endothelial cells of the veins express attachment factors which encourages the coagulating and clotting of blood and development of thrombus. Sickle-cell anemia, which can cause blood cells to cluster up and block veins, can likewise prompt stroke. Stroke is the subsequent driving reason for death in individuals under 20 with sickle-cell anemia. Air pollution may likewise increase stroke risk.

EMBOLIC STROKE

An embolic stroke refers to an arterial embolism (a blockage of an artery) by an embolus, a traveling debris or molecule in the arterial circulatory system originating from somewhere else. An embolus is most frequently, yet it can likewise be various different substances including fat (e.g., from bone marrow in a broken bone), air, disease cells or bunch of microorganisms (generally from infectious endocarditis).

Because an embolus emerges from somewhere else, nearby treatment tackles the issue just temporarily. Accordingly, the main source of the embolus should be identified. Since the embolic blockage is abrupt from the onset, symptoms are normally maximal at the beginning. Likewise, symptoms might be transient as the embolus is somewhat resorbed and moves to an alternate area or dissipates altogether.

Emboli most usually arise from the heart (particularly in atrial fibrillation) however may begin from somewhere else in the arterial tree. In perplexing embolism, a deep vein thrombosis embolisms through an atrial or ventricular septal deformity in the heart into the brain.

<u>*Reasons for stroke connected with the heart can be distinguished between high and low-risk:*</u>

High Risk: atrial fibrillation and paroxysmal atrial fibrillation, rheumatic illness of the mitral or aortic valve sickness, artificial heart valves, known cardiovascular thrombus of the atrium or ventricle, sinus syndrome and disorder, sustained atrial flutter, recent myocardial localized necrosis, ongoing myocardial dead tissue along with ejection fraction <28% percent, congestive cardiovascular failure with ejection fraction <30% widened cardiomyopathy, Libman-Sacks endocarditis, Marantic endocarditis, *infective endocarditis, papillary fibroelastoma, left atrial myxoma and CABG(coronary artery by-pass graft) surgery.*

Low risk/potential: calcification of the ring (annulus) of the mitral valve, PFO (patent foramen ovale), atrial septal aneurysm, atrial septal aneurysm with patent foramen ovale, left ventricular aneurysm without thrombus, isolated left atrial "smoke" on echocardiography (no mitral stenosis or atrial fibrillation), complex atheroma in the proximal arch ascending aorta.

Among the individuals who have a total blockage of one of the carotid conduits, the risk of stroke on that side is around 1% for every year.

A unique type of ESUS (embolic stroke is the embolic stroke of undetermined source). This subset of cryptogenic stroke is characterized as a non-lacunar brain infarct without proximal cardio embolic sources or arterial stenosis. Around 1 out of 6 cases of ischemic stroke could be diagnosed or classified as ESUS.

CEREBRAL HYPOPERFUSION

Cerebral hypoperfusion is the decrease of blood flow to all parts of the cerebrum (brain). The decrease could be to a specific part of the brain contingent on the cause of it. It is usually because of cardiovascular breakdown (heart failure) from arrhythmias or cardiac arrest, or from decreased cardiovascular output because of myocardial, aspiratory infarction, pericardial emission, pulmonary embolism, or bleeding.

Hypoxemia (low blood oxygen content) may boost the hypoperfusion. Since the decrease in blood flow is all over, all pieces of the cerebrum (brain) might be affected, particularly vulnerable "watershed" regions. A watershed stroke is a condition when the blood supply to these regions is compromised. Blood flow to these areas doesn't really need to stop, however, it might decrease or lessen to a point where cerebrum (brain) damage happen.

VENOUS THROMBOSIS

Cerebral venous sinus thrombosis leads to stroke because of locally increased venous tension or pressure, which surpasses the pressure produced by the veins or arteries. Infarcts are bound to go through hemorrhagic change (leaking of blood into the harmed region) than different types of ischemic stroke.

INTRACEREBRAL HEMORRHAGE

It by and large happens in small arterioles or arteries and is regularly due to hypertension, intracranial vascular mutations (this includes cavernous angiomas or arteriovenous distortions), cerebral amyloid angiopathy, or even infarcts into which secondary hemorrhage has occurred. Other possible causes are bleeding problems and disorder, amyloid angiopathy, trauma, drug abuse, for example amphetamines or cocaine. The hematoma broadens until strain and pressure from surrounding tissue restricts its growth, or until it de-pressurizes by emptying into the ventricular system or the pail surface. 33% of intracerebral bleed is into the cerebrum's ventricles. ICH has a death pace (mortality rate) of 44% after 30 days, higher than ischemic stroke or subarachnoid hemorrhage (which in fact may likewise be categorized a kind of stroke).

Other different other causes may be spasm of an artery. This might due to cocaine

SILENT STROKE

Silent stroke is stroke that has no outward or physical signs and symptoms, and individuals are usually uninformed they had experienced stroke. In spite of not causing recognizable and identifiable symptoms, silent stroke actually damages the cerebrum or brain and spots the individual at high risk for both transient ischemic attack and major stroke even in the future. On the other hand, the people who have had major stroke are likewise in danger of having silent stroke.

In an expansive report and examination in the year 1998, about more than approximately 11 million individuals were estimated to have experienced stroke in the US. Around 770,000 of these were symptomatic and 11 million were very first silent X-ray infarcts or hemorrhages. Silent stroke regularly causes injuries which are recognized through the use of neuroimaging like X-ray. Silent stroke is estimated to occur 5X the pace of symptomatic stroke. The risk of silent stroke gets worse with age, yet they may likewise affect more youthful adults and kids, particularly those with acute anemia.

CHAPTER THREE
DIAGNOSIS &
PREVENTION

Stroke is diagnosed through a few methods and techniques: a neurological examination (like the NIHSS), CT checks (most frequently without contrast enhancement) or X-ray scans, Doppler ultrasound, and arteriography. The analysis and diagnosis of stroke itself is clinical, with help from the imaging methods. Imaging method additionally help with deciding the subtypes and cause of stroke. There is yet no generally used blood test for the stroke diagnosis itself, however blood tests might be of help in figuring out the probable cause of stroke in deceased individuals, an autopsy of stroke might help laying out the time between the start of stroke and demise.

PHYSICAL EXAMINATION

A physical examination, including taking a clinical/medical history of the signs and symptoms and a neurological status, helps giving an assessment, evaluation and estimation of the area and seriousness of stroke. It can give a precise and standard score on e.g., the NIH stroke scale.

Here is an example of what it looks like (although medical practioners will understand this better):

Imaging

For diagnosing ischemic stroke in an emergency position or setting:

CT scans (without contrast improvements or enhancement)

Specificity= 96%

Sensitivity= 16% (under 10% in initial 3 hours of symptom).

X-ray scan:

Specificity= 98%

Sensitivity= 83%

For diagnosing hemorrhagic stroke in the emergency position or setting:

CT scans (without contrast improvements or enhancements);

Sensitivity= 89%

Specificity= 100 percent

X-ray scan

Sensitivity= 81%

Specificity= 100 percent

Note: *For identifying chronic hemorrhages, an X-ray check is more sensitive.*

CT scans may not identify ischemic stroke, particularly if it is small, of onset, or in the brainstem or cerebellum regions (posterior infarct). X-ray is better at identifying a posterior circulation infarct with diffusion-weighted imaging. A CT scan is used more to preclude specific stroke mimics and to identify bleeding. The presence of leptomeningeal collateral circulation in the cerebrum is related with better clinical results after recanalization treatment.

Cerebrovascular reserve capacity is one other factor that affects stroke result - it depends on how much increase in cerebral blood flow after a purposeful stimulation of blood by the doctor, like by giving inhaled carbon dioxide or intravenous acetazolamide. The increase in blood flow can be estimated by PET or transcranial Doppler sonography. Nonetheless, in individuals with impediment of the inner carotid vein or artery of one side, the presence of leptomeningeal circulation is related with decreased cerebral reserve capacity.

HIDDEN AND UNDERLYING CAUSE

At the point when stroke has been diagnosed, different examinations might be performed to decide the hidden and underlying cause. With the ongoing treatment and diagnosis options available, it is of particular significance and importance to determine if there is a peripheral source of emboli. Test selection might differ since the reason and cause of stroke changes with age, comorbidity and the clinical presentation. These are the usually and common used methods:

i. *An ultrasound/Doppler examination of the carotid arteries (to identify carotid stenosis) or dissection of the prevertebral veins,*

ii. *An electrocardiogram (ECG) and echocardiogram (to identify arrhythmias and resultant clumps in the heart which might spread to the cerebrum (brain) vessels through the circulatory system),*

iii. *A Holter monitor examination to identify irregular strange or abnormal heart rhythms,*

iv. *An angiogram of the cerebral vasculature (if a bleed is thought to have started from an aneurysm or arteriovenous mutation),*

v. *Blood tests to decide whether blood cholesterol is high, in the event that there is an unusual tendency to bleed, and if a few processes, for example, homocystinuria may be involved.*

For hemorrhagic stroke, a CT or X-ray scan with intravascular contrast might have the option to identify irregularities or abnormalities in the cerebrum arteries (like aneurysms) or different sources of bleeding, and structural X-ray in the event that this shows no cause. On the off chance that this also doesn't identify a fundamental justification for bleeding, invasive cerebral angiography could be performed yet this requires access to the circulation system with an intravascular catheter and can create additional stroke as well as further complications at the insertion site and this examination is consequently reserved for a very specific situation. On the off chance that there are symptoms proposing that the hemorrhage could have occurred because of venous thrombosis , CT or X-ray venography can be used to study or examine the cerebral veins.

MISDIAGNOSIS

Among individuals with ischemic stroke, misdiagnosis occurs 2-26% of the time. A "stroke chameleon" (SC) is stroke which is diagnosed as another thing else.

Individuals not having stroke may likewise be misdiagnosed with the condition. Giving thrombolytic (clot busting) in that kind of case makes intracerebral bleeding 1 2% of the time, which is not exactly that of individuals with stroke. This pointless treatment adds to the medical care costs. However, the AHA/ASA rules and guidelines express that starting intravenous tPA in potential mimics is liked to postponing treatment for extra and additional testing.

Women, African-Americans, Hispanic-Americans, Asian and Pacific Islanders are more frequently misdiagnosed for a condition other than stroke when as a matter of fact having stroke. Furthermore, adults under 44 years old are multiple times bound to have stroke missed than are adults over of 75 years old. This is particularly the situation for younger individuals with posterior infarcts. A few medical centers have used hyper acute X-ray in exploratory and experimental examinations for individuals initially thought to have a low probability of stroke, and in a portion of these individuals, stroke has been found which were then treated with thrombolytic medication.

PREVENTION STARTEGIES

The most effective way to assist with preventing a stroke is to eat a good and healthy diet, work-out regularly, and try not to smoke or drink in excess.

These lifestyle pattern can decrease your risk of issues like:

Hypertension and High blood pressure

Veins and arteries becoming obstructed or clogged with fatty substances (atherosclerosis)

High cholesterol levels

If by any chance you already had stroke, making these changes and improvements can assist with reducing your risk, chances, and possibility of having another later on i the future.

1. DIET

An unhealthy eating meal and diet can increase the possibilities and chances of having a stroke since it might prompt an increase in your circulatory strain and cholesterol levels.

A low-fat, high-fiber diet is suggested and recommended, including a lot of fresh fruit (say 5X Every Day) and wholegrains.

Guaranteeing an equilibrium and balance in your eating regimen is extremely important. Don't eat a lot or too much of a single food, especially food varieties high in salt or processed food sources.

You ought to restrict how much salt you eat to something like 6g (0.2oz) a day as a lot of salt will increase your circulatory strain (blood pressure): 6g of salt is around 1 teaspoonful.

2. EXERCISE AND WORKOUT

The combination of a healthy diet and regular exercise is the most effective way to keep or maintain a healthy weight.

Standard and regular exercise can likewise assist with bringing down your cholesterol and keep your blood pressure sound.

For a great many people, no less than 150 minutes (2 hours and 30 minutes) of moderate-intensity aerobic activities, for example, cycling or quick strolling.

Doing it consistently is what i would suggested.

On the off chance that you're recuperating or recovering from a stroke, you ought to examine and discuss possible exercises with the individuals from your recovery and rehabilitation group/team.

Making exercise a custom may not be imaginable or possible in the first weeks or months after a stroke, however you ought to have to start exercising once your recovery process has advanced and progresses.

3. QUIT SMOKING

Smoking fundamentally builds your risk of suffering a stroke. This is on the grounds that it limits your arteries or veins and makes your blood bound to clot and cluster.

You can likewise your risk of having a stroke by stopping smoking.

Not smoking will likewise work on your overall health and lessen your risk of having other difficult conditions, like heart disease and cancer of the lungs.

The National Smoke free Helpline is willing offer consolation and encouragement to assist you with stopping smoking. Call 0300 123 1044 (England specifically).

4. ELIMINATE LIQUOR AND ALCOHOL

Excess consumption of alcohol can prompt hypertension (high blood pressure) and trigger a sporadic heartbeat (atrial fibrillation), the two of which can expand your risk of suffering a stroke.

Since alcohol are high in calories, they likewise cause weight gain. Weighty drinking duplicates the risk of stroke by more than 5X. So assuming you decide to drink liquor or alcohol and have completely recovered, you ought to do whatever it takes not to surpass the recommended limits.

I often advise individuals not to drink up to 14 units in a week. So spread your drinking over 3 days or more if it's possible that you drink as much as 14 units every week

If by any chance you have not completely recuperated or recover from your stroke, you might find out that you have become delicate and sensitive to alcohol and, surprisingly, the *recommended limit point might even be a lot for you.*

CHAPTER FOUR
RISK FACTORS AND DIET

The main modifiable risk factors for stroke are hypertension and atrial fibrillation even though the size of the effect is little; 833 individuals must be treated for 1 year to prevent 1 stroke. Other modifiable risk factors are:

- ☐ *High blood cholesterol levels,*
- ☐ *Diabetes mellitus,*
- ☐ *End-stage kidney disease,*
- ☐ *Active and Passive cigarette smoking*
- ☐ *Weighty alcohol use,*
- ☐ *Drug use,*
- ☐ *Absence of physical activity,*
- ☐ *Processed red meat consumption, and lastly*

☐ *Unbalanced and unhealthy diet.*

Smoking only 1 cigarette each day heightens the risk more than 30%. Alcohol consumption could incline toward ischemic stroke, as well as intracerebral and subarachnoid hemorrhage by means of different systems and mechanisms (for instance, by means of atrial fibrillation, rebound thrombocytosis and platelet collection, hypertension, and coagulating disturbances).

Medications and drugs, most usually amphetamines and cocaine, can prompt stroke through damage to the veins or blood vessels in the brain and acute hypertension.

Headache (Migraine) with aura multiplies an individual's risk for ischemic stroke.

Untreated celiac disease no matter the presence of signs and symptoms can be a hidden and underlying cause of stroke, both in young individuals and adults. In regards to the 2021 WHO study, working 55+ hours, 7 days, raises the risk of stroke by 35% and the risk of death from heart conditions by 17%, when contrasted with a 35-40 hours week.

High degrees of physical activity lowers the risk of stroke by around 26%. There is an absence of top notch examinations and studies taking a deep look at promotional endeavors to further develop and improve lifestyle factors. Regardless, given the huge collection of proof and evidence, best clinical management for stroke includes counsel on diet, exercise, smoking and use of alcohol. Medicine is the most well-known technique and method for stroke prevention; carotid endarterectomy can be a valuable and useful surgical method for forestalling (preventing) stroke.

PULSE AND BLOOD PRESSURE

Hypertension accounts for 35-50% of stroke risk. Decrease in blood pressure of 10 mmHg systolic or 5 mmHg diastolic lowers the risk of stroke by ~40%. Lowering down circulatory strain (blood pressure) has been definitively shown to prevent both ischemic and hemorrhagic stroke. It is similarly significant in secondary prevention. Even individuals older than 80 years of age and those with disconnected systolic hypertension benefit from antihypertensive therapy. The already available evidence and proof doesn't show much contrasts and differences in that frame of mind between antihypertensive medications — in this manner, different factors, for example, protection and immunity against different types of cardiovascular sickness and cost ought to be considered. The standard routine use of beta-blockers keeping stroke or

TIA has not been displayed to result in benefits.

BLOOD LIPIDS

High cholesterol levels have been conflictingly related and associated with (ischemic) stroke. Statins have been proved to highly reduce the risk of stroke by around 15%. Since prior Meta examinations of other lipid-lowering drugs didn't show any decreased risk. Statins could apply their effects through components and mechanisms other than their lipid-lowering effects.

DIABETES MELLITUS

Diabetes mellitus gradually increases the risk of stroke by 2-3 times. While concentrated and intensive glucose control has been displayed to decrease small blood vessel or vein difficulties and complications, for example, kidney damage and also damage to the retina of the eye and it has not been displayed and shown in order to bring down huge vein intricacies and complications', for example, stroke.

ANTICOAGULATION DRUGS

Oral anticoagulants, for example, warfarin have been the pillar of stroke prevention for more than 50 years. In any case, a few examinations have shown that aspirin and other antiplatelet are profoundly compelling and effective in optional counteraction after stroke or transient ischemic attack. Low dosages of aspirin (for instance 75-150 mg) are essentially effective as yet make less symptoms; the lowest effective dose until date remains unknown. Thienopyridines (clopidogrel, ticlopidine) may be somewhat more successful and effective than aspirin and have a less developed risk of gastrointestinal bleeding, yet are more expensive.

Both clopidogrel and aspirin might be valuable at first few weeks after a minor stroke or high risk TIA. Clopidogrel has less incidental effects than ticlopidine. Dipyridamole can be added to aspirin treatment to give a little extra advantage, despite the fact that migraine (headache) is a typical side effect. Low-dose aspirin is likewise more effective for stroke prevention subsequent to having a myocardial infarction.

Individuals with atrial fibrillation have a 5% a year risk of stroke, and this risk is higher in those with valvar atrial fibrillation. Relying upon the stroke risk, anticoagulation with prescriptions, for example, warfarin or aspirin can be very useful for prevention with different degrees of relative viability depending on the sort of treatment used. Oral anticoagulants, particularly Xa (apixaban) and thrombin (dabigatran) inhibitors have been demonstrated to be better than warfarin in stroke decrease and have a lower or comparative bleeding risk in patients with atrial fibrillation. Besides individuals with atrial fibrillation, oral anticoagulants are not recommended for stroke prevention — any advantage is balanced by bleeding risk.

In essential and primary prevention, antiplatelet drugs will not decrease the risk of ischemic stroke yet increase the high risk of major bleeding. Further examinations are needed to explore a potential defensive effect of aspirin against ischemic stroke in women.

SURGERY

Carotid endarterectomy or carotid angioplasty can be used to eliminate atherosclerotic narrowing of the carotid corridor. There is proof supporting this technique in few selected cases. Endarterectomy for an important stenosis has been demonstrated to be valuable in forestalling and preventing further stroke in the people who have previously had the condition. Carotid artery stenting has not been shown and proved to be similarly useful. Individuals are selected for a surgery based on age, orientation, level of stenosis, time since symptoms and the individual's preferences.

Surgery is most proficient when not delayed for too long— the risk of repetitive or recurrent stroke in an individual who has a 50% or more, stenosis is up to 20% after 5 years, but endarterectomy lessens this risk to around 5%. The number of procedures expected and needed to cure 1 individual was 5 for early surgery (in not less than about fourteen days after the initial stroke), but 125 whenever delayed longer than 12 weeks.

Evaluating and screening for carotid artery narrowing has not been proved to be a helpful test in the general population. Examinations of surgical processes for carotid artery stenosis without signs and symptoms have shown just a little decrease in the risk of stroke. To be valuable and beneficial, the complexity pace of the surgery ought to be kept under 4%. And still, after all that, for 100 surgeries, 5 individuals will benefit by preventing stroke, 3 will foster or develop stroke regardless of the surgery, 3 may die due to the surgery itself, and 89 will remain stroke-free yet would likewise have done as such without intervention.

DIET

WHAT YOU NEED TO BE AWARE

- *After a stroke it very well may be harder to get every one of the supplements or nutrient you need.*
- *Your speech pathologist can prescribe methodologies or strategy to help you eat and drink.*
- *Your dietitian can assist with ensuring that you are getting sufficient and adequate nutrition.*
- *Good and healthy dieting can greatly improve or lessen your risk of having another stroke.*

ABOUT POOR NOURISHMENT

- o *After a stroke, you might have:*
- o *Issues using your arm or hand, making it challenging to eat and drink.*
- o *Issues with memory and thinking, which could mean you can easily forget to eat and drink.*
- o *Loss of craving and appetite - you may not feel hungry.*
- o *Swallowing issues, which are likewise called dysphagia.*

These challenges might make it hard to get every one of the supplements and nutrient you need. This can slow down your recuperation.

Assuming that you have issues with your arm or hand, or with your memory and thinking ability a medical specialist or therapist can assist with techniques and Aids to assist you with remembering all. If by any chance you have dysphagia, a speech pathologist can prescribe techniques to help you eat and drink safely.

IMPROVE YOUR DIET

A dietitian can assist with ensuring you are getting adequate nutrition. This might mean having specific kinds of food and drinks, eating pretty much food and taking healthful and nutritional supplements.

RULES FOR A HEALTHY

DIETING

1. *Fruits*

o *A lot of vegetables of various colors and types, beans, and legumes.*
o *Grain (oat) foods, for the most part are wholegrain and contain high fiber like cereals, rice, bread, pasta, noodles, polenta, quinoa and barley, couscous, and oats.*
o *Lean meats and eggs, tofu, poultry, seeds, fish, nuts, vegetables and beans.*
o *Milk, yogurt, cheddar and their other options - usually reduce fat level.*
o *Drink a lot of water.*

2. *Limit consumption of food varieties containing Sugar, added salt, and saturated fats:*

o *Limit food sources high in fat, for example, cakes, pastries, biscuits, pies, burgers, processed meats, pizza, potato chips, fried foods, crisps, butter, cream, cooking margarine, coconut oil and palm oil.*

- ○ *Limit food varieties and drinks containing added salt.*
- ○ *Limit food varieties and beverages containing added sugars for example sugar sweetened soda pops and cordials, vitamin waters, fruit drinks, sports drinks and energy drinks.*

HEALTHY DIETING AFTER STROKE

Vegetables and fruits contain antioxidants, which can assist with reducing damage to veins. They additionally contain potassium which can assist with controlling blood pressure.

The fiber in fruits and vegetable lower cholesterol. Folate - (which is usually found in green green-leafy vegetables) - may lower the risk of stroke.

Cereals and Wholegrains additionally contain fiber and folate.

Dairy food sources are one more source of potassium, alongside calcium, which can likewise assist with controlling blood pressure. Options in contrast (alternatives) to dairy include calcium-enhanced soy or rice milks.

Different sources of calcium are fish with bones, tofu and almonds.

Things to restrict from after stroke are:

    I.   *Salt.*

- *An excessive amount of salt can raise your blood pressure. Understand or read labels and pick lower salt options.*

- *Try not to add salt while cooking or at the dining table.*
- *Instead, use spices and herbs to increment flavor.*

In the event that you decrease your salt consumption gradually, consistently, and continuously, your taste buds will adjust in a matter of time.

II. Sugar.

- *An excessive amount of sugar can damage blood vessels.*
- *Pick lower sugar options.*
- *Indeed, even food varieties you may not consider sweet can have added sugar.*

III. Soaked fats.

- *These causes high level cholesterol.*
- *Eat for the most part polyunsaturated and monounsaturated oils and*

spreads. You can also try avocado or nut boarders.

CHAPTER FIVE
CAREGIVERS GUIDE

If you were hired to be a caregiver, in order to do an exquisite job, you must see the patient and victim as a loved one or family. That is the only way you can do a great job and that is how i will address that person as throughout the whole chapter: "as a loved one".

Stroke recovery can be confusing and troublesome for survivors. This chapter is intended to assist you, as a caregiver, in better ways with navigating the recovery process, social and financial aftermath of a stroke. I have provided tricks and tips on how to best communicate with the medical care team and deal with stroke's effects, as well as data on legal assets, health coverage, and info legal resources.

BASIC EMOTIONAL SUPPORT

Shock, vulnerability, worry, helplessness, and stress are normal among stroke survivors and their friends and family. Just after a stroke, it's typical as usual to feel emotional and uncertain about your new job as a guardian or caregiver — maybe in light of serious and severe constraints or changes of personality in your loved one. You could likewise worry and try to anticipate another o stroke and that it's your obligation and duty to prevent that.

Truth be told; at this junction, your relationship with your loved one has additionally been adjusted. Other than your past obligations or responsibilities, you might need to take on additional house hold chores that your loved one used to handle.

To assist you with acclimating to your new obligations, this segment will guide you in finding the emotional support you really need from your local friends, family, and community.

By expanding your knowledge about what stroke is and what you should expect, you can feel less overwhelmed and have more control. So this is what i suggest you do:

*• **Ask more questions;** what kind of stroke is your loved one having? What side of the cerebrum (brain) is affected? What even caused the stroke? To what level did it affect your loved ones capacity? What are the preventive measures to take to prevent another one?*

*• **Do all necessary research**; it's very possible to beat stroke and rehabilitation is critical to accomplishing victory on the way to recovery. On this journey, you will have*

to make many choices and be an advocate for your loved one.

• Get more knowledge on the effects of stroke; *Each and every stroke is interesting and unique, so knowing the effects of the stroke on your loved one will definitely assist with posing the right inquiries of their medical care team.*

• Look for more info on caring for a stroke survivor; *Call the Stroke Family Warm line to talk with our trained experts who can give various helpful info, interface you to local services or on the other hand be a listening ear. You can likewise request a packet of info to be sent to you via email in light of your particular or specific need. (1-888-478-7653) or Stroke.org/SpeakWithUs.*

REQUEST FOR SUPPORT/HELP FROM OTHERS

- ***Connect and reach out to friends, and loved ones;*** *Let them know what you are experiencing. Make telephone calls, messages or some other common time can yo quite far to assist you with feeling supported and restored.*

- ***Build a network with other caregivers and stroke survivors;***

- Month to month Stroke Connection e-news gives more info and motivation to caregivers and stroke survivors. In it, you'll find more info and updates on conditions that might prompt stroke, for example, hypertension, as well as the physical, behavioral and communicative conditions stroke might cause. It too offers tips for everyday living and supportive info for

guardians and caregivers. You can join at (StrokeConnection.org).

- Join a support group: Recovering from a stroke, or really caring for somebody who is, can be emotional. Being there for one another is the reason i have lunched a virtual support community for stroke and coronary illness survivors and their families.

- Assist with coordinating and organizing a stroke support group or reinforce a current one in your local area. Visit Stroke.org to learn more about starting a care/support group.

• Think about seeking professional assistance*; Pastoral counselors and Mental Health Professionals can pay attention to your various questions while showing you adapting abilities.*

GET CALCULATED/ACTIVE HELP AND SUPPORT

Giving care to a stroke survivor can rewarding. Yet, it tends to be distressing and baffling when you're abruptly pushed into a caregiver role. That is a difficult position. It's among life's most difficult jobs, as a matter of fact. There's frequently little and brief period to plan.

In the event that you've quite recently became a caregiver, remember this: To succeed, you should deal with your necessities and needs as well as the survivor's.

*• **Build A Supportive System;** Characterize and define precisely the things you really need, request help on representative obligations, for example, meals, shopping for grocery, Hospital visits, yard work, and so on.*

- Pen down the things that are generally too hard for you to do and search for the ideal individual for the gig.

*• **Also prioritize and Focus on your time**. You might have other different roles and obligations beyond being a caregiver, for example, being worker, parent, wife or husband, or local area pioneer (community leader). It's vital to continue to find balance for you as well as your immediate family (incase the stroke victim is not).*

CARVE OUT TIME FOR YOURSELF

• Eat a well-balanced diet; Figure out how you can keep up with great dietary patterns that help prevent stroke and coronary illness (heart diseases).

• Get regular physical activity.

• Carve out time to enjoy a hobby maybe once per week.

• Invest time with your loved ones (that includes friends).

• Begin writing a journal. Journaling can assist you with alleviating pressure, put together your thoughts and spend some time all alone.

CLLINICAL MANAGEMENT

Speaking with the health care group can assist you with understanding what occurred during your loved one's stroke, what you should expect during the recovery cycle and how to support recuperation and recovery. This can assist you with feeling less anxious and overpowered.

You should provide the Health care Group with a detailed Medical history such as:

• Allergies

- *Past illness or diseases*

- *Medications*

- *Family History*

- *Surgeries in the past*

REHABILITATION

Rehabilitation is very critical and basic to many stroke survivors' healing. The best level and percentage of recovery as a rule happens in the first year after a stroke, in spite of the fact that it could go on for years — especially if victims keep pressing on the areas they want to improve. In any case the speed of recovery after the first year is probably going to extensively sluggish and slow.

Recovery can assist with further developing stroke survivors' freedom and independence in numerous areas, that includes taking care of oneself, communication skills, mobility, and mental and social abilities and skills. Under a specialist's guide, rehabilitation experts give a treatment program intended for the stroke survivor's requirements and needs.

Caregivers assume a fundamental part in stroke survivors' recovery. Caregivers ought to get some information from the health care team about recovery or rehabilitation services immediately to guarantee your loved one is headed toward recovery quickly. Then you can converse with the medical team and rehab group about how you can assist with recovery at home, also in any case help with your loved one's individualized recovery plan.

Recovery services Might Include:

• *A Diet and Nutritional care*

• *A Speech, language, cognitive or hearing therapy*

• *An Occupational therapy*

• *A Physical therapy*

• *Rehabilitation nursing*

• *Sporting treatment*

• *Recovery counseling*

• *Social work*

• *Mental or psychological treatment (for instance, post stroke discouragement)*

• *Chaplaincy*

• *Support groups*

• *Professional and vocational assessment*

• *Driver's preparation*

• *Projects and programs to work on physical and emotional strength in order to get back to work.*

MAKE A FIRST AID PACK

In case of an emergency, be ready to give health care professionals essential documents and information. Store them in a protected location. Tell your relatives as well as close friends where they are hidden. Download a complete rundown of emergency docs at caregiverstress.com.

<u>*Here are list of what an emergency kit contains:*</u>

• Rundown of key contacts (doctors, family individuals, and so forth.)

• Rundown of drugs, including portions and frequencies

• A copy of your loved one's health insurance card(s)

• A copy of the clinical development directive.

LEGAL FINANACIAL AND HEALTH

As a new caregiver, getting a grip on lawful, monetary and medical problems can be overwhelming. This section will motivate & kick you off.

Priorities straight: Assemble key health and legal docs your loved one has created or could need to update. These include:

• Advance mandate (living will) — A patient's open and clear statements of wishes about their medical services. This maintains a strategic distance from questions and disputes about treatment choices and provides guidance to medical care suppliers. To get to state-specific advance directive structures and instruction, visit the

United States Advance care Plan Registry.

• Last will and confirmation — determines who will get an individual's assets upon death. This likewise achieves different targets, including naming guardians for minor children or youngsters.

• Overarching legal authority (the power of attorney) — appoint someone else to make financial and legal decision.

• HIPAA Rep form — HIPAA (The Health Insurance Portability and Accountability act form specify who can have access to an individual's classified or confidential medical info.

MONETARY AND FINANCIAL ASSISTANCE

Stroke recovery and rehabilitation can be expensive, even when a patient has good health coverage. But compounded with loss of work, these can deplete family funds. Check out these resources that might be useful to ease the strain:

• Converse with the specialists and experts.

- Social specialists can assist you with exploring private and government handicap and insurance programs. Social worker are available at most clinics and rehabilitation facilities and can be located by calling 1-800-677-1116.

– Certified financial planners and legal practitioner specialized in elder care and disability can also be useful.

• AARP Money Management Programs — Everyday money management services are responsible for helping older, disabled, or low-income people who have financial hardships.

• AARP Tax-Aid — helps and assist with giving help with completing tax documents for people age 50 or older.

MEDICAL COVERAGE

• *Understand your ongoing or current health care*

• *Consider acquiring health care insurance if not done yet or if necessary*

- Call the health care insurance company. Figure out what services will and won't be covered and what recovery and rehabilitation administrations are available.

- On the off chance that the health care insurance company won't pay for your loved one's care, on a second thought, you can file a petition/appeal.

- The Health care Insurance Commercial center, lunched as a feature or part of the affordable

Care Act in 2014, gives access to health insurance option with a standard set of benefits.

- Acquiring health care insurance can be really challenging. Counsel the

Patient Advocate Foundation free direct advocacy services, including help with getting health care and getting health insurance and solving medical debt issues.

CHAPTER SIX
JESUS THE WAY OUT

There's one more way out of Stroke: The way is called Jesus!

There's no infection, be it terminal that God can't heal. Despite what has held you down, Jesus speaking In Matthew 11:28 " Come to me, all you that are burdened and are heavy laden, and I will give you rest. Convey my weight upon you, and learn from me; for I'm simple in heart: and you will find rest in your spirits. For my weight is incredibly simple, and my weight is light."

Regardless the circumstances you are going through Jesus can help you if you have faith in him.

Anyway, to do that, you must receive him into. If you are yet to receive Jesus Christ, say this:

"Dear Jesus, I know that I am a sinner. I recognize that you died on the cross for my sins and rose again in light of my justification. Henceforth, I acknowledge you as my personal savior and lord. Likewise, I proclaim and declare that the power of Satan, Sin, Death and Hell is broken over my life for I'm in Christ now. So be it!"

The most extraordinary miracle is going to happen in light of the fact that you believe and have faith in him. Trust God with your healing and every other issue.

The following are a couple of scriptures that could be useful to you;

Isaiah 38:16-17, Isaiah 57:18-29, Jeremiah 33:6, Isaiah 40:29, Matthew 11:28, Jeremiah 30:17... .. Run to Jesus now!!!

Essentially in the event that you truly need direction, connect with me one on one through this mail - will394560@gmail.com

www.ingramcontent.com/pod-product-compliance
Lightning Source LLC
Chambersburg PA
CBHW070820280726
48660CB00017B/2149